How to Pass A Drug Test for Marijuana

The Ultimate No B.S. Guide for How to Beat A Drug Test

Table of Contents

Introduction

Today's version of the internet has many articles and products that promise to make you pass a drug test with little to no research on your part. However, in order to pass a drug test, you must take the time to learn the techniques, how they affect your body, and how drug tests actually work.

It is also crucial to learn what techniques are not actually proven to work and what techniques have been proven to work by science. By learning these, you can begin to take all the steps needed to stack the odds in your favor for the next drug test you are going to take.

It also must be stated that there is no 100% guaranteed way to pass a drug test, despite the numerous publications that promise such things. The truth is, you can take certain steps to ensure you have the best chance in passing a urine drug test, but you can never do a one-step guaranteed action that will eliminate all possibility of failing a test.

The first step in ensuring that you have the best chance to pass your test is to learn about how the creatinine levels in your blood affect your urine concentration. Also, it is important to learn the problems and risks with water dilution. It is a myth that drinking tons of water the night before a test is the optimal way to dilute your urine. This has not been scientifically backed and causes a lot of misconceptions for people looking for the easiest and most truthful techniques to use.

It is recommended that you take notes while you are reading this short and concise book. This will ensure that you get the most out of the information in here. The notes will help you to pinpoint exactly what you need to implement and by writing things down, you will be able to recall specifics and how to handle certain situations when they arise.

Lastly, remember that everything in this book has been compiled through evaluating the latest research, so feel free to question what you have read in this book. It is encouraged that you conduct your own research on the topics, concepts, and techniques that you want to look even deeper into.

It is also worth mentioning here that there are many websites on the internet offering discussions, forums, and experiences where you can learn a lot on this matter. Some even offer products that can help you pass the test. All will ultimately depend on your own personal judgment since the information in this book will only serve as a guide.

The more you understand about your own blood, urine levels, and the processes in your body, the better off you will be. To pass an upcoming drug test, it will take some preparation, planning, and work on your part but you can tilt the odds in your favor! So remember to read with confidence and an open mind!

Chapter 1:

Drug Tests - An Overview

In the fast-paced world that we live in, many people will do almost anything to land a job. This includes the tedious process of fine-tuning the appropriate application documents needed, putting in the necessary financial means, and this may or may not include drug testing.

Various employers have their own reasons for setting up drug tests in their job application process, ranging from liability reductions to plain insurance cost cutting. Even the Federal Government mandates every business establishment to be clean of drug-related blemishes before they can ever get their hands on a business contract, and before actual work commences.

Why Are Employers Promoting Marijuana Drug Testing?

There are several reasons why employers mandate job applicants, as well as current employees, to undergo marijuana drug testing. The decision is only practical for many. Some of these reasons are:

They want to maintain or enhance productivity. Employees who are not dependent on marijuana tend to be more productive in workplaces. They accomplish much more work compared to frequent marijuana users.

They want to assist in the community. If a community approaches a particular employer for assistance of any kind, the management with sincere concern for its employees' well-being may provide assistance.

They intend to deliver a message against drug use. If an employer is a serious, well-respected and dominant figure in a particular industry, he/she usually must promote serious employment as well. This includes the proper management of a workplace and its employees.

They intend to contain health care concerns. Employers prefer to control health care concerns of their employees. Some take the initiative of extending financial assistance to their people. Since different health complications can be associated to marijuana users, it is a practical move for them to hire "clean" employees.

They prefer to rehabilitate employees. If they want to maintain or improve the workplace, a marijuana test can help them identify employees who are in need of rehabilitation.

Additionally, a marijuana drug test is often seen as mandatory in a workplace, since it promotes the health and safety of employees and clients.

However, there are still a few commercial establishments that can be considered "drug-test free". As the size and number of employees in these establishments increase, so does the responsibility of ensuring the integrity of their workforce. This includes ensuring chemicals such as metabolites don't hamper their employees' productivity and work ethic.

With this in mind, it is also worth mentioning that the possibility of certain drug-screening procedures affecting the productivity of employees is there; and the vast majority of employers still think that the only way effective employment processes can be truly taken to the next level is to employ clean drug-testing procedures on their premises.

Common Drug Testing Types

There are also restrictions on the employer's end as to when, how, and why drug testing should be put into order. One is that employers must do drug screenings to test for drugs - the law forbids the testing of other illnesses or medical situations during drug tests.

This seems to shed light on the importance of knowing just how long substances included in drug testing remain in one's body, which will be tackled in a later chapter.

The term "drug testing" may consist of the following forms:

Hair Testing

Hair testing for marijuana is a popular type of drug testing. The popularity is due to three main reasons: the results are almost impossible to adulterate, subjects are unable to do a quick "clean up", and the results allow an extended look-back period.

Usually, a standard hair testing procedure requires 1.5" of hair (preferably head hair). It is reliable since signs of marijuana ingestion show in the hair follicles. The signs remain almost indefinitely. Even marijuana ingestion that occurred a year ago is identifiable with hair testing.

Oral Fluid-Based/Saliva Drug Screens

If marijuana was consumed within the past 12 to 24 hours, an oral fluid-based/saliva drug screens can detect it. This is an easy and effective way of testing marijuana ingestion. The results are very difficult to spoil as well.

The particular procedure resembles that of a blood test procedure. After the acquisition of a saliva sample, it is sent to a lab for analysis.

For this reason, oral fluid-based/saliva drug screens are a favorite among employers with the available funds. This enables them a quick, non-invasive, and easy pre-employment solution.

Blood Tests

Blood tests for the recognition of marijuana usage are very accurate. The aim is to point out an actual substance, instead of just metabolites. As mentioned, these tests are similar to oral fluid-based/saliva drug screens.

A concern with blood tests for marijuana use is its detection time. It is relatively short. For a user that ingested marijuana once, 3 to 4 days is the notable detection time. For a frequent user, detection time is generally less than a week.

Sweat Drug Screens

Since sweat contains a chief ingredient in marijuana called *THC* (or Tetrahydrocannabinol), sweat drug screens are a precise way of detecting marijuana consumption.

Its success is primarily dependent on appropriate sample collection. The procedure usually begins with a patch application on the skin. After 10 days, the patch is sent to a laboratory for analysis.

Sweat drug screens are effective in detecting marijuana in the system. They can present complicated results, however. This is mostly due to the effect of temperature and various environmental conditions on the sample amount of perspiration.

Testing for Anabolic Steroids

With the popularity of marijuana in the anabolic steroids cluster comes the increasing popularity of testing procedures for marijuana ingestion for anabolic steroid users. The majority of the subjects are fitness trainers, bodybuilders, and athletes.

Urine Drug Screens

Urine drug screens are another popular test for marijuana usage. It can detect the ingestion of marijuana for up to 5 days (infrequent users). For those who are chronic users, it can detect for up to 30 days.

The test is very effective. Given, however, the fact that people have unique metabolic rates, the duration of the tests can vary quite a bit.

In the event that a user takes particular pharmaceutical medications, the results of urine drug screens can report a false positive. Some of these drugs are *Ibuprofen, Naproxen, Promethazine, and Sulindac.*

Other Marijuana Drug Screening Types

Another type of drug testing is called *random screening*. Random screening is the one with the most controversial methods, and opposition is so strong that some states like Rhode Island and California (to name a couple) have come up with their own countermeasures, which put a restriction on screenings in private places, in order to prevent unjust procedures.

There is also a test called *The Duquenois-Levine Regeant*. It is a screening test especially established for marijuana detection. Since its initial development in the 1930s, it gained recognition worldwide for being one of the most effective methods for cannabis drug testing. Due to its effectiveness, it was adopted by the United Nations in the 1950s. It is essentially a chemical color reaction test. To guarantee unbiased results, a 3rd party administrator is usually involved.

The process begins by creating a special solution, which is added to dried petroleum, hydrochloric acid, and chloroform. Then, another chemical is used. If the chemical turns into a purplish hue, the presence of marijuana is indicated.

Chapter 2:

Knowing the Substance

Some of the most well-known and common situations when drug tests are performed are post-accident, random, pre-employment, return-to-duty, and reasonable suspicion testing. Of these, random drug testing might be the most stressful experience any drug user will ever have.

Random drug testing is stressful because not every individual feels comfortable at the thought of getting tested. Imagine your name being called out of 100 employees unexpectedly. The incident can make you panic if you have any uncertainty about your recent recreational or medicinal behavior. Regardless of innocence with regard to drug use, you still might feel as if you are in trouble.

A Look on General Drug Tests

Since most employers will most likely not perform testing procedures during times that negatives results will be likely, a majority will test employees when they least expect it. In this procedure, the employee to be tested is almost always "machine-picked", using computer software capable of numbering in random, with the quantity of employees addressed by the employer.

This increases not only the chances of an employee's name getting picked more than once, but really impacts the stress levels as well. Before delving deep into the procedures, it is important to have the appropriate knowledge-base of what's being tested and how it affects the body.

The most commonly used drug-screening procedures, like the 10 panel urine sample screening, tests for the following substances: Barbiturates, Amphetamines (including Methamphetamine), Buprenorphine, Cannabinoids (THC), Cocaine, Opiates (Codeine, Heroin, Morphine, Oxycodone, and Hydrocodone, among others.), Methadone, Propoxyphene, Methaqualone, Phencyclidine (PCP), Benzodiazepines, Tricyclic antidepressants, Synthetic Cannabinoids (K2, Spice).

One of the important factors to understand prior to undergoing a drug test is the drug test detection times and the duration of certain kinds of substances in one's body. Detection times for different substances depend on various factors such as metabolic rates, body mass, amount and frequency of use, age, health conditions, and urine acidity.

Marijuana as the Focus

In the case of marijuana, the detection time is determined by the half-life of the substance Tetrahydrocannabinol. The half-life of Tetrahydrocannabinol, which is the active ingredient of marijuana, is 10 days. Metabolism plays a large role in determining detection times with different users.

Aside from the factors already mentioned above, detection times also depend on other factors such as:

Body Type

For those with relatively more body fat than average, marijuana detection takes less time. Since the components in marijuana are fat-soluble, marijuana consumption is easier to recognize in the system.

Marijuana use is certainly recognizable in skinny people as well. However, with lower body fat, the results can take a while to process.

Tolerance

A marijuana user's tolerance level affects detection times. The system of those with low tolerance for marijuana will most likely show minimal indications. In this case, their body prefers to eliminate the substance immediately.

Conversely, those with high tolerance levels will show signs of marijuana in their system faster. Within a day, it is usually identifiable. Even if the consumption occurred more than a year ago, signs may remain detectable.

Marijuana Potency

Detection times are also influenced by the potency of marijuana. If the substance has apparent effects on a user, detection tends to be relatively faster. This is due to the active benefits of marijuana in his system.

On a related note, recently prepared marijuana is more potent than the earlier marijuana. Most likely, if the user ingests a freshly rolled joint, detecting marijuana in his/her system will only take 12 to 24 hours.

Method and Frequency of Marijuana Use

Frequent marijuana users (almost daily marijuana users) can easily detect signs of marijuana in their system. Since the substance does not exit immediately in a frequent user's body, indications will be obvious within 24 hours.

The method of marijuana use is also a factor. The list of common methods of ingestion include: *smoking, vaping, skin application (topical products), eating edible marijuana, and drinking tinctures.*

Most likely, if marijuana is in the system, the use is detectable faster. Depending on the type of marijuana test, internal indications of marijuana can be revealed within a month.

If marijuana is absent inside a system, detection times tend to be longer. Signs of skin applications of marijuana may take longer and be more difficult to detect. In some cases, detection is impossible.

Fluid Intake at Time of Test

Marijuana use is easier to detect with moderate fluid intake at the time of testing. Conversely, for a user who consumes more fluid than necessary, detection may be slower.

This factor also addresses the type of fluid taken within moments of marijuana testing. If the fluid in subject is water, detection can be accomplished faster. In cases of alcohol, energy drinks, unique juices, and different fluids with strong chemicals, detection times can be delayed. This is due to the possibly complex effects of the fluids within the body.

Exercise Frequency

With irregular exercise sessions, detection times for marijuana use tends to be processed quickly. This is compared to users who frequently exercise.

The variation in time is due to the marijuana inside the system. If a user exercises frequently, the components in marijuana can exit the body through perspiration.

Patient's Condition

A patient's condition affects detection times for marijuana use, since some marijuana users have health complications. This is because these illnesses can delay the recognition of the substance inside the system.

Gathering More Information on Marijuana

It is also suggested to be familiar with marijuana as a substance. This way, you can have a hint of its influence on the body for such procedures.

While marijuana is one of the most popular drugs, not a lot of people are thoroughly informed on the full effects of it. It has quite a variety of physical and psychological effects.

In most cases, the effects of marijuana start minutes after inhalation, and the effects can last for hours. Compared to inhalation, its effectiveness when ingested (via eating or drinking) can take a bit longer.

What About the Marijuana High?

The effects of marijuana are usually referred to as *the marijuana high*. It has short-term and long-term influences on the body. Popularly, it is known to make a user experience visual and auditory highs.

Potential Physical Effects of Marijuana:

Dry mouth

Rapid heart rate

Tingling sensations

Hunger and thirst

Red tongue

Cracked lips and soreness in mouth

Glazed eyes

"Munchies" (or appetite increase)

Potential Psychological Effects of Marijuana:

Low inhibitions

Silliness

Dissociative personality episodes

Giddiness

Sleepiness

Paranoia

Anxiety

Chapter 3:

Knowing the Methods

Another crucial step is to know the different methodologies used in testing individuals for drugs. The basic methods are through saliva, hair, blood, and urine. Carefully deciding on which of the four methods to use beforehand is crucial and therefore this must be decided cautiously.

With every job hunt should come the responsibility of checking out applicable local state laws, knowing your basic applicant's rights, and the awareness that certain laws on hiring practices (including discrimination) exist and will help make the job search easier.

Methodologies via Accredited Sectors

It is suggested to undergo marijuana use testing in an accredited testing center. The teams behind accredited testing centers have undergone rigorous training. According to industry standards, their methods are effective.

Accredited testing centers are also reliable. For a first timer, the complexities of methodology preferences of particular testing centers are rather questionable. The fact that a testing center is accredited enhances confidence. Regardless of the failure to understand concepts entirely, they are more likely to follow through.

Method # 1:

Gas Chromatography

The first one we will talk about is *Gas Chromatography*. In this procedure, urine samples are divided into its component parts inside chromatographic columns. This is done by inert gases onto which individual boiling points for each column help determine the affinity of the extracts.

Individual retention times help in compound identification and are unique for each drug in a given procedure. By observing recommended retention times, the procedure tends to be a success.

A downside of Gas Chromatography for marijuana use testing is the long finalization period. In a few cases, a single sample has to undergo analysis for more than an hour. To serve as a follow up procedure, additional time is necessary.

Typically, it is an effective method for the detection of marijuana use. It does, however, require multiple testing for confirmation.

Method #2:

Immunoassay

Our second method is called *Immunoassay*, which is used to determine solubility by using complex substance mixtures. Urine and serum, for example, are biological fluids containing analytes. In turn, these analytes are used together with antigen-antibody tests in finding illegal substances.

Its success is dependent on particular factors. One of these factors gives light to back-up laboratory equipment. For laboratories that are rather extensive, Immunoassay may be useful. However, for a small laboratory, it may only bring unnecessary expenses.

This procedure, despite having a few recorded false positive results, is 97-99 percent accurate. In the event of one, failure is usually blamed on improper sample handling rather than on the procedure itself. Due to its effectiveness, it is a method often used in analytical chemistry and forensic science.

Generally, Immunoassay's effectiveness as a biochemical test addresses the presence of a small molecule in a small solution. With this small molecule's detection comes the recognition of a protein.

Immunoassay is presented in various formats. Sometimes, it necessitates the use of a calibrator. This allows for faster completion of the entire procedure.

Moreover, it is based on the principle that highlights the complex nature of molecules. One of its goals is to define a measurable signal. Therefore, it is not an impossibility for it to link chemicals with a detectable label.

Testing with Regard to Accuracy

Testing through saliva, as with any oral fluid-based screening, gets its accuracy from the ability to detect just a few days use of illegal substances and is therefore one of the methods highly chosen by experts due to being adulteration-proof and convenient.

Performed usually by the employers themselves, and due to the fact that various intoxication degrees can be determined by the amount of drugs in one's system alone, oral tests are a highly-preferable method for both post-accident and on-the-job drug abuse situations.

Needless to say, accurate results are important. If the results are rather misleading, the process of marijuana testing turned out to be a waste of time for all parties involved. While those who are attempting to beat the system find this to work in their favor, it can trigger a re-test – and an unexpected one.

Expensive Tests: Are They Worth Paying?

On the subject of expensive testing for marijuana detection, the service exchanged is usually justified. Those who have prepared funds are usually satisfied with the results and experience peace of mind.

Many employers allot a budget for marijuana testing primarily because marijuana testing is cost effective. While there are some who prefer the least costly solutions, other employers insist on relying on accurate results above all.

So far, the most expensive way of testing for illegal substances is through blood. And because it's expensive, it's also the least common. While it is regarded as the most accurate of all the methods, it is also the most intrusive.

Hair testing on the other hand is another expensive testing method for marijuana use. It makes use of the natural tendencies of THC to be deposited into the hair. This is possible by accessing blood vessels in the head for its testing accuracy.

Tetrahydracannabinol stays permanently in the hair, and the test consists of extracting them by dissolving hair samples in different types of solvents. However, this method has its drawbacks, ranging from the inability of some laboratories to discriminate split hair samples even from the same donor, to declining to test drug history greater than your average hair growth.

Getting away with this method is also exceptionally difficult. As it turns out, some of the workaround proves too much. There is a chance that some strategies will only damage your hair permanently.

This is because THC has the tendency to stay in your body for weeks. However, on an average cost of a few dollars more than the urine test, the results can be solid.

Chapter 4:

Masking Techniques That Do and Don't Work

Many marijuana users refuse to give up marijuana consumption entirely, even if they must be tested for some reason. Instead, they continuously find ways to beat the system. In this day and age, some techniques are known to be successful.

With the rise of the internet, an increasing number of discussions are relayed. Surprisingly (to some), masking techniques are not disregarded. As it turns out, more and more people are contributing to discussions about marijuana masking.

For someone who is trying to pass the test, it is best to be informed of the factors that can help their chances. It is also equally important to know the factors that can lead to further trouble.

Why Resort to Masking?

Marijuana users resort to masking techniques in order to pass testing. Especially if they know the testing date is approaching, the scheduled techniques help them conceal marijuana use. A person can use them for a quick way of redemption.

Before even trying out hearsay, knowing what does and doesn't work will allow a person a higher chance to beat the tests.

Masking the Smell: Hiding Identifiable Odors

The smell of marijuana is unmistakable, especially for examiners. It is distinguishable due to its strength.

Avoid tactlessness when going in for a marijuana drug test. It can make examiners suspicious, and consequently, subject you to further doubts. Any indication of marijuana with you points to the fact that you are a marijuana user.

Wash your hands. If you held a stash of marijuana for a friend, clean your hands thoroughly.

Masking Techniques That Do NOT Work

While it is a fact that some masking techniques don't guarantee complete eradication of the substance from the body, some actually work to mask marijuana traces in the urine; and there are still other masking methods that do more harm than good. Dilution techniques are a good example of these.

6 Ineffective Masking Techniques:

1) Among those that do not work is the masking agent *Goldenseal*. While some testified it did wonders for them, it doesn't. Scientifically it hasn't proven to make a significant difference for those looking to pass a urine drug test.

Yet, laboratories are presuming adulteration if you have excessive amounts of the masking agent in your system, due to the fact that so many still use it despite failing to achieve beneficial results.

2) Taking Zinc Sulfate, which is actually passed as stool rather than waste from your bladder, is another way to fail your drug test. Niacin, like Goldenseal, also won't help. The same holds true with Puri-blend products. All of these have been said to help hide traces of marijuana use,

however, the science does not back up these products or the chemicals used in them.

In fact, masking marijuana use with zinc sulfate, niacin, and Puri-blend products hold dangers. The technique can be toxic. It can cause blood sugar abnormalities, liver failure, nausea, vomiting, and heart palpitations.

3) Another very important thing to consider is never to add anything (including water) to your specimen just to aid in passing the tests. Specimens like urine have specific gravity factors that are easily altered and can be specified as ground for adulteration.

4) A masking technique rumored to work is taking aspirin, which is said to interfere with assaying and help yield negative results, but many modern laboratories have adapted and are able to work around this testing flaw - leaving this technique useless in most up-to-date testing centers.

Taking aspirin needlessly also triggers adverse effects. The list of these effects includes nausea, stomach pain, ulcer, blood loss, gastritis, heartburn, cramps, headaches, and rashes.

5) It is worth clarifying here that drinking gallons of sports drinks, tea, cranberry juice, or even water prior to testing won't do you any good. As stated earlier, flushing THC entirely from your body within a few hour period is virtually impossible as far as drug testing is concerned.

Matters become more complicated when random testing is taken into consideration, making the likelihood of a positive result fairly high.

6) Do not overload on water the few days prior to your test because this will dilute your creatine levels and electrolytes for the test. Most up-to-

date testing centers can pick up on this and have adjusted to people using this loophole in the past.

This is a huge misconception which many people fall victim to because of being misinformed. They try to load up on water the day before the test to dilute their urine, when in actuality, they are diluting their creatinine levels to an extreme amount and this appears to be very suspicious to the people looking at the results.

Masking Techniques that DO Work

Three Potentially Effective Masking Techniques:

1) Discontinue the use of over-the-counter medication for 90 days. Skip the chance to use analgesics since these can influence the effects of marijuana, and leave hints of the synergy. For a pre-determined period, rely on natural treatment alternatives.

Additionally, the discontinued use of medications will make it easier for your system to eliminate signs of marijuana. Due to the absence of medications' side effects, regulated body processes are dependable.

2) Detoxify with detox supplements. These products are very effective in flushing out

marijuana, among all toxic chemicals in the system. They can be used to flush out almost every trace of the drug.

Usually, the supplements for detoxifying your system in preparation for marijuana testing require use for a pre-determined amount. To guarantee the products' effectiveness, a marijuana user should avoid unhealthy habits as well.

3) Creatinine levels play a major role in the dilution process. Raising one's creatinine levels - which is a creatinine byproduct after being metabolized by the body for 48 hours - from the normal range of about 110-200ng/dL will help to lower the chances of getting a positive result on the test. The aim is to normalize creatinine levels. A figure around 0.2 means normal creatinine.

Elevating creatinine levels is a good technique for masking marijuana use. However, it is not always suggested since elevated creatinine levels is an indication of impaired kidney function. Here are some ways to raise your creatinine levels:

Foods

Consume foods that are rich in protein during the week prior to the test. Foods such as green, leafy vegetables, lean chicken, beef, and steak will all help to raise creatinine levels. Lean steak is especially helpful with providing creatine to the body.

Supplements

Taking an iron supplement for the weeks prior to a test can be a great idea as well. It will help to ensure that you have strong iron levels in your blood because a lowered iron level will decrease your urinary creatinine levels.

Creatine supplements can help as well but make sure that you are only taking up to 5mg a day. Keep in mind that creatine loading is only a good strategy when you prepare at least 2 weeks in advance. It takes around a week for the creatine to load up in the bloodstream.

Exercise

Exercising for around 30 minutes a day in the few weeks prior to a drug test will help excretion. Do not do anything too strenuous in a desperate attempt to pass your test. People have tried to do over-the-top workouts the days before a test and it hasn't shown to make any significant difference according to the scientific studies. You will be better off just exercising a little each day then run 15 miles the day before your test.

Vitamins

Some vitamins can also be used in conjunction with other dilution techniques in order to help you achieve better results. B2 and B complex vitamins helps urine retain its yellow color by taking at least 2 to 3 each morning, while making sure any "old" THC-loaded urine in your system has already been flushed out. Be sure to consult with your doctor in regards to vitamin supplementation!

Chapter 5:

Passing the Test & Swapping Samples

Sometimes, drastic times may call for drastic measures, and one possible drastic measure screeners will take in exchange for a negative result is urine substitution.

Substituting one's urine sample against a synthetic one is a very risky procedure and offers just three possibilities should a person get caught: current job loss, future job opportunity loss, and worse: jail.

What About Special Cases?

Drug testing in special cases of probation/parole are usually carried out instantly at the office of the officers in charge. While it may be true that Parole Officers usually only monitor the whole procedure without observing, it is no excuse to be well cleansed of the substance in question.

It is better to be on the safe side and make sure you're virtually toxin-free before taking the tests. It is also the best way to veer away from all the stress the situation might cause you.

Employees must also take note that employers are also obliged to provide a special documentation of observed behavior in the advent of a suspicion that you are using alcohol or prohibited drugs at work. The document must be detailed and well documented before they can even send you for tests based on reasonable suspicion.

Here are additional tips worth reading that can help you beat your tests:

Bring proper identification, including government-issued ones like military IDs, passports, driver's license, etc. When taking marijuana tests, it is basic protocol to be ready with such proof of identification. With the presence of these IDs, a representative from the employer is no longer necessary.

Turn your cell phone off while the tests are ongoing. It's beyond good manners to tend to your phone relentlessly while a collector is attending to you. It will also raise suspicion if the phone goes off while you are in the testing process.

Listen and pay special attention to the instructions that the collecting officers tell you. If you have questions, don't hesitate to ask. By listening to the instructions carefully, you can find loopholes to buy time, if you need it.

Go alone and don't bring someone along if possible, for there's a big chance they won't be allowed even inside the testing premises.

Be punctual. If you are on time for your drug testing, it will leave an impression that you're eager to pass the test and won't raise suspicion on behalf of the collecting officer.

One of the most important documents of a drug test is the Custody and Control form. It is an official record containing information about your Medical Review Officer, the name of the collector, exact testing location, and specimen ID and data.

Respect for the Examiner

Many people give the excuse to the collecting officer that they are unable to urinate at the time of the test and hope to use this as an excuse to not take the test at all. Depending on the rules in place for your specific test, the collecting officer will most likely have one of two rules they enforce.

You will either have to schedule another time to take the test in the very near future, or you will have to stay on the testing premises until you are finally able to go.

However, experienced examiners are aware of such an excuse. He/she may observe you for indications of attempts to outsmart them. If the examiner gets the message that you are disrespecting his/her authority, you may be penalized. Consequently, you are attracting trouble instead of cutting yourself some slack.

If you respect and treat your collecting officer accordingly, everything else will fall in place. The rules are quite simple and merely revolve around courtesy. Be punctual, follow every instruction, and deliver your specimen appropriately. Humility and goodwill will go a long way.

Talking to Laboratory Agents

An observed screening is one done with strict supervision from the experts behind the testing and is called upon for a number of reasons, like testing via court orders, military service, past tests that have failed, or as simple as your specimen failing to meet their criteria.

Sometimes, the top eligibility for an observed test is specimen substitution/tampering and negotiating with the sample collector can be next to impossible. With this in mind, caution and "practice" must be considered, contrary to approaching your testing unprepared.

If the decision to approach the people in laboratories for help is final, make sure to do it responsibly. Remember, not many laboratories accept this behavior. It can result to an offense, and worsen punishment. Moreover, a list of important reminders is shown below should you decide to take the substitution route.

Switching Urine Samples: What You Need to Know

Urine can still be good for a year as long as it's sealed in an airtight container and frozen. Specimens kept for shorter periods need less refrigeration time - usually a week. Urine specimens kept under room temperature can last for a couple of days even without refrigeration.

Take note that synthetic urine comes in 2 basic forms:

Liquid Type - can be found in smoke shops; used for lab equipment calibration

Powder-Concentrated Vials - can be added to water

Keeping Samples Warm

It is important to submit warm samples. Ideal specimen temperatures can be achieved either by using a hand-warming sporting device to warm the specimen container or by simply warming it on a glass of hot beverage.

It is very difficult to come up with approximate numbers on when a pot smoker would test clean, since so many "interconnected" factors are at play here. The safest way is to test your very first daily urine output (at least twice a week, since this is usually the average detoxification time of an average smoker) until it tests clean.

Besides detecting marijuana, the procedure also tests for metabolites - the byproducts of marijuana, after it has gone through the body's systems that collect in the urine.

More Tips:

Make sure your specimen and everything you need for beating the drug test is good and dependable. In the case of substitution, make sure your synthetic urine (or any other urine for the particular purpose) is prepared for the timing of the test. Practice makes perfect. And in this part, home tests and validity strips can be your friends. They can be bought at leading drugstores near you or even over the internet.

Avoid buying brand new products that promise to guarantee unrealistic results. If you take a product and fail the test, oftentimes it will look even worse to the evaluator because it will seem as if you tried to cover up your traces along with using the marijuana itself. To avoid this, always make sure to research the chemicals and ingredients placed in a new product.

Since collectors will be on alert for any unusual noises posing a threat to the procedure's integrity, always make sure you can have access and will be able to quietly open your container in whatever place is safe for you to do the switching.

You should transfer your synthetic urine immediately upon finding the right moment inside the restroom. Court-deployed and simple employment testing usually don't require the use of gowns.

Urine samples coming from immediate family members and/or friends can be kept somewhere safe in your clothing for up to 12 hours as long as the samples are clean.

In case of a predicament wherein the collector obliges to put the gown immediately upon your arrival at the office or lab premises, prepare an excuse that you really need to go to the restroom badly. Pity from the testing staff should give you plenty of time to switch samples and prepare yourself.

You should never attempt, at all costs, or even try to inject synthetic urine directly into your bladder to avoid the risks associated with infections. This is often done under pressure. If a marijuana user is desperate, the technique will be used.

Be absolutely certain to keep your synthetic samples from your examiner's eyes. In the event of deterioration, the examiner might become suspicious, and rigorously monitor you.

Human digital thermometers can also be a big help when using this method. This guarantees that the urine stays at normal body temperature.

A well-cleaned, pocket-sized shampoo container taped securely in your crotch can be a safe way to store your synthetic urine. Well-rinsed, non-lubricated condoms can be used with the shampoo bottles to keep it warm inside, say, your crotch for example.

It has been regarded that the best place to keep your samples warm is right between your scrotum and anus, where the sample can be kept at a constant 94-95 degrees.

As additional points of advice, relying heavily on predictions from software and/or various graphs and charts can be useless due to inaccuracy. Most laboratories indicate "50 nanograms of THC/milliliter" as a conjectural positive.

Crossing your legs while sitting down (with the sample container between your thighs) can even raise the sample temperatures to 97-98 degrees.

One technique specifically for women is placing their synthetic samples in unsuspicious places such as placing two 1-oz containers on each breast with the support of a well-padded bra. Body heat in their chest ensures warmth of the urine sample.

The vaginal cavity can also be a good place where the sample can be kept at a stable 98 degrees. Since it is a hollow structure, it can provide sufficient space for the urine sample.

Chapter 6:

Where to Test

While testing facilities are popping up all over the place, the most common locations for random, follow-up, return-to-duty, or pre-employment tests are at hospitals, medical clinics, laboratory facilities, or simply on the employer's premises - if sufficient equipment is available.

Less strict employers let employees on their screen lists make arrangements with the sample collection facilities at their own convenience. Pre-employment collection facilities usually don't send representatives from the employers to supervise the testing. It is therefore the sole obligation of the employee to be punctual and responsible for his or her own testing procedures.

DERs, or Designated Employer Representatives, can be deployed by some employers especially in cases such as return-to-duty, reasonable suspicion, follow-up, or random testing where the law itself decides on such deployments. This ensures the integrity of the results by eliminating possible adulterations and other tampering of the samples to achieve negative results.

ISO 17025: What Is It?

ISO (or International Organization for Standardization) first issued ISO 17025. It is meant to be a standard for testing laboratories and calibrations worldwide. Testing centers with an ISO 17025 demonstrate technical competency.

Sometimes, ISO 17025 is referred to as *IEC* 17025 (or International Electro technical Commission). It is suggestive of accreditation via voluntary review process.

A laboratory with an ISO 17025 certification means it has quality management systems. According to the certification, its operations undergo a thorough evaluation regularly. The assessment is done regularly to guarantee progressive technical competence and compliance with industry standards.

For an employer with serious objectives of getting employees and applicants tested, approaching centers with an ISO 17025 certification is best. While they can charge relatively more expensive fees, some testing centers with the particular accreditation provide quality services.

Testing Centers & Their Adherence to Laws

It is important to undergo marijuana testing at a center that complies with laws. Usually, the laws vary by state. The need to set laws is for controlling the number of testing centers.

A basic law that the operators of testing centers should follow is to maintain integrity in the industry. Their motive should not be corrupt and it should not revolve simply around money.

After all, it is not difficult to establish a testing center. Acquiring capital, as a primary step, can be done. Unfortunately, there are groups who open testing centers, run tests, and distribute unsupported results.

The Need for a COE

A Conditional Offer of Employment, or COE, is sometimes bundled by employers in their onsite testing procedures to help motivate employees to pass the tests and land the jobs. Onsite employee testing is carried out usually in two ways.

One, a company may be hired by employers to send sample collecting officers to the testing site. Two, your company has employees trained specifically to perform the testing. Pre-employment tests are unlikely after two to three weeks of landing the job but it is important to be reminded that it can still be deployed randomly, so it is sometimes safe to use illegal substances after one's first paycheck.

Possible Problems in Testing Centers

Sometimes, regardless of a testing center's competence, problems with marijuana use detection arise. It can present unquantifiable results. Especially if the laboratory has been operating for a while, its practices might be outdated. Consequently, it can only provide estimated figures, instead of precise ones.

It is important for a testing center to use valid methods. It should eliminate traditional practices and inaccurate formulation. Invalidated methods for chemical analyses cannot guarantee quality results.

Moreover, it is a requirement for testing centers to have a reference standard. With one, they can yield precise results, and proceed with quality operations.

List of Potential Problems

Lack of Experience

Inexperienced people in testing centers might yield wrong results due to improper calibration settings. Since laboratory equipment can work in varying resolutions, improper calibration can provide results – results that are not maximized.

Refusal to use Conversion Strategies

Avoid testing centers that disregard conversion strategies. Their argument may be because conversion is unnecessary. For them, only if an imbalance is identified should the need for conversion come up.

However, there's a high chance of their unreliability. Contrary to their claims, conversion factors are necessary for pointing out exact measurements. One popular conversion factor is *decarboxylation conversion factor*. Testing centers should not ignore this factor since it allows accurate calculations.

Residue Buildup

During the repeated analyses of samples for marijuana testing, residues can build up. This can also be due to lack of cleaning. The result is highly exaggerated laboratory results.

Sometimes, residue buildup is called *ghost peaks*. The origin of the term addresses the needlessness of residues.

Testing Centers Management

An on-site chemist should manage a particular laboratory testing. He/she should hold a PhD in chemistry (or in a relevant industry). He/she should also possess 8 years of experience to ensure he can handle typical and candid requests. The professional's full-time presence indicates the reliability of a testing center.

With a chemist, you can ask for assistance every step of the way. Since he/she understands chemical properties and reactions, he/she can provide detailed discussions.

Chapter 7:

The Results

Regarding results, it is unfortunate that as an applicant, you may never get your hands on your drug test results; but as an employee, you have every right granted by law to see your results.

This can be done via special request from the HR Department, which will in turn give you a detailed copy of the results. In the event of testing positive, an interview with the MRO in charge of your testing is inevitable and therefore you must be armed with enough knowledge of the possible reasons of the results, especially in the case of a false positive.

The Credibility of the MROs

Most Medical Review Officers are true to their work, and while they can never be an integral part of the lab, the fact that they get their paychecks straight from the employers is enough to make justifying illegal substance use, by tears or by words, very difficult.

In the first place, it will be an insurmountable task to justify the presence of illegal substances in your body because of the absence of any legal reason behind it.

On the other hand, if you should take a stand against a positive result from a legal point of view, the proficiency records of the finished testing can be reviewed via subpoena from your lawyer.

The whole process may involve a number of processes. This is to ensure quality in marijuana use testing. Usually, respectable authorities in the marijuana industry oversee this process.

Most quality control measures of a vast majority of laboratories are updated and reviewed if any need arises. Remember that these laboratories are staffed with incredibly skilled professionals. The occurrence of discrepancies in their practices is unlikely but possible.

An Insider Look at Laboratories

A large majority of laboratories go through proficiency testing on a regular basis. A sign of the ongoing developments in marijuana laboratories is the insistence to undergo proficiency testing.

While their reputation says their operations are already effective, they welcome possible improvements. This step is laudable, and is a sign of growth in facing different challenges in the marijuana industry.

For the most part, proficiency testing addresses the effort of promoting *quality assurance*. Given the fact that the marijuana industry is a fast-growing industry, operations are updated regularly to guarantee honest services.

Periodic blind specimen laboratory submissions are carried out. These specimens may be positive, negative, adulterated, or substituted. For status confirmation, they should acquire certification from suppliers. Alongside, they should come with supplier-established expiration dates.

Both negatively and positively confirmed samples are forwarded. Negative specimens especially, necessitate verification by accepted methods. The verification can be accomplished via Gas Chromatography or Immunoassay.

In case of adulterated specimens, the protocol suggests that the status should still be certified. If possible, it should also be confirmed. If any of these submitted specimens are found to be "out of the ordinary", the lab's license might be revoked.

Guaranteed Quality

Ensure that testing is undergone through an accredited laboratory. Accreditation suggests competence, and it guarantees the establishment of analyzed methods.

ILAC (or International Laboratory Accreditation Cooperation) serves a prominent role in guaranteeing that testing laboratories are effective. It inspects a particular laboratory, and it meticulously examines this laboratory's operations.

Moreover, an accredited laboratory is a representation of a well-structured laboratory. Accreditation conveys the message that it follows protocols and meets industry-standard requirements.

Among these requirements are:

Proficiency testing should include all items within a laboratory's scope.

Third-party administrators of proficiency testing should have accreditation.

Proficiency testing should reveal numerical accuracy.

Personal Role in Final Testing Phase

While their competency remains in mind, many laboratories encourage subjects to ensure flawless marijuana use testing. This privileges you to inform a laboratory of your submission. Alongside, it allows you to specify that a blind specimen should be distinguishable from an ordinary specimen.

While the teams from laboratories can provide services, as well as assistance when necessary, it is up to you to ensure successful testing.

Duties:

You should guarantee that the specimen-collector adheres to protocols. Check whether he/she places initials on specimen bottles.

You should guarantee that submitted blind include a variation of split specimens.

You should submit blind specimens according to a laboratory's rules and regulations.

Accepting the Results

In the event that you submitted contrary to expected results, accept the findings. If you tested positive for marijuana consumption, you know whether the result is just. The same goes if you have tested negative and your preferred result is positive. You always have the option to question the results.

As the practice of laboratories go, it is more practical to conduct 0 tests, instead of providing inaccurate or misleading results. With a reputation to uphold, the accredited laboratories are very thorough with their operations.

Questioning your test results can be an expensive process and a time-consuming one too. The MRO's duty of collecting, reviewing, and analyzing lab test results to ensure the integrity of the results is a job relying entirely on facts.

If you are taking other medications that might have triggered your positive result, it is also their duty to contact the pharmacies/physicians involved to make sure the prescriptions are addressed to the right person. As all possible angles are deemed for investigation.

Any mismatch from the lab reports down to the amount of THC in your urine will just place an accent to your positive findings. If you smoke pot, you should therefore be well aware that THC, along with its metabolites, could stay in your body for weeks.

www.ingramcontent.com/pod-product-compliance
Lightning Source LLC
Chambersburg PA
CBHW070547290526
45790CB00002B/600